Eosinophilia:
Fast Focus Study Guide

JT Thomas, MD

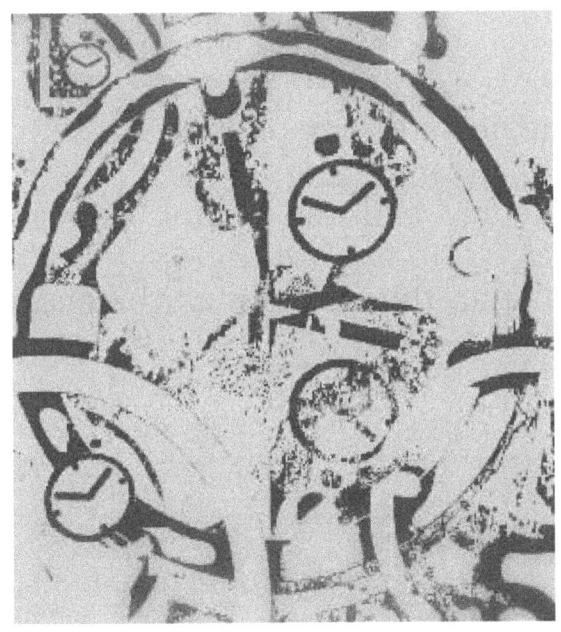

Acknowledgements

I dedicate this book to my beautiful wife and children, who I love more than all the water in all the oceans and all the seas.

CONTENTS

- This book is written to help the reader further understand the causes and diagnosis of Eosinophilia.

- This book is written in a simple and easy to read format designed for medical students, residents and physicians who are preparing for boards.

- This book simplifies a complicated medical issue so you will remember the important details.

- You will not get caught up in the minutia. Just the facts are found in this book.

- This Fast Focus Study Guide will provide you with a practical review of the key information you need to know.

- Buy this book now if you want this quick and concise information

The diagnosis of Eosinophilia can be placed into into 3 big categories.

I: clonal (or primary) eosinophilia

II: reactive (or secondary) eosinophilia

III: idiopathic hypereosinophilic syndrome (HES).

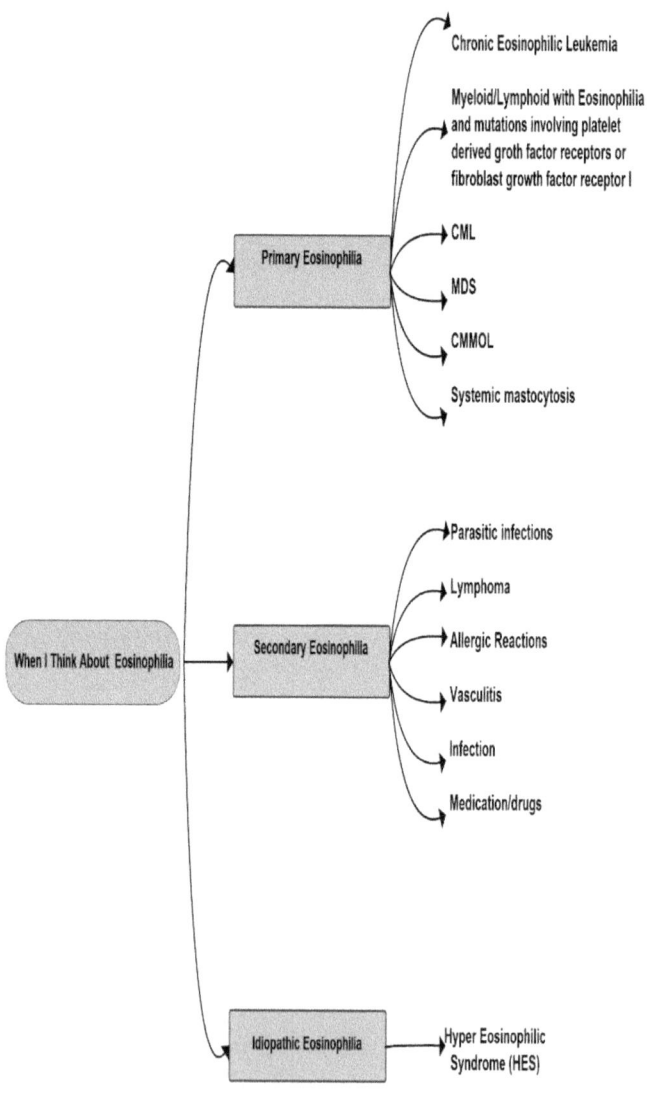

Normally we first think about reactive (secondary) eosinophilia. Secondary causes of eosinophilia are things like infection or allergic reactions.

Primary eosinophilia (clonal eosinophilia) is typically part of a myeloid malignancy or occurs as a manifestation of a clonal disease characterized by a cytogenetic or molecular genetic marker.

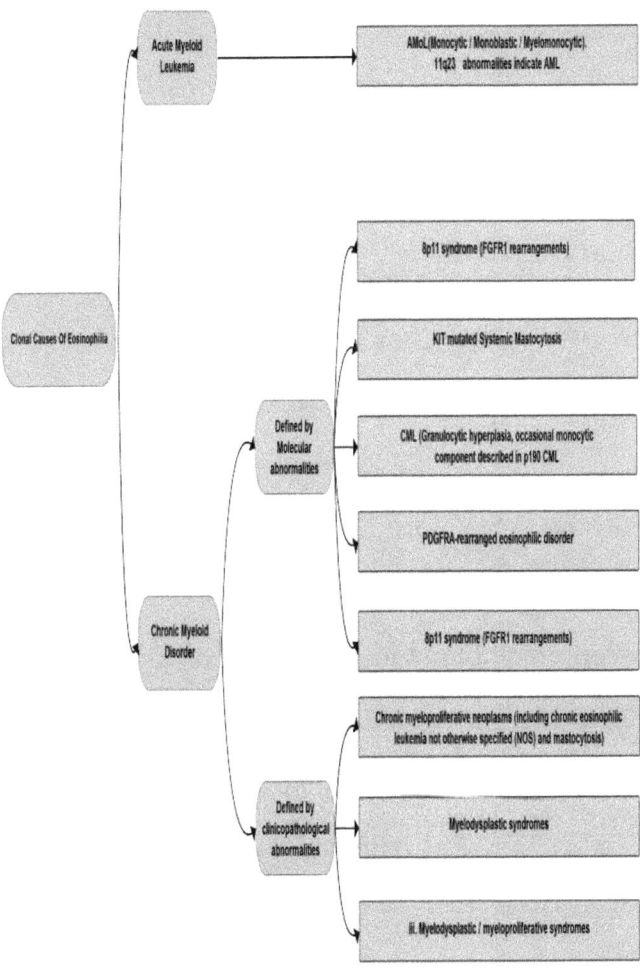

When checking for primary (Clonal) causes of eosinophilia we are going to perform the following tests.

-Bone marrow aspirate and biopsy

-Cytogenetics on bone marrow aspirates.

-Peripheral blood for molecular analysis for FIP1L1-PDGFRA fusion gene

-Peripheral blood for Molecular analysis for Wilms tumor (WT) gene.

-Peripheral blood for evaluation of tryptase and decreased erythropoietin as well as demonstration of JAK2 which could indicate presence of a myeloproliferative disorders.

What are we looking for in the bone marrow?

We might see acute leukemia.

We might see myelodysplasia.

We might see a myeloproliferative disorder.

The bone marrow will be stained for reticulin fibers looking for myelofibrosis.

We will stain for tryptase looking for a mast cell disorder.

Flow cytometry will be done looking for CD 52 and CD 117.

What are we looking for in the bone marrow
cytogenetics?

We might see 5q33 (PDGFRB)

We will be looking for 8p11 (FGFR1)

Samples will be tested for FIP1L1-PDGFRA fusion
gene either with FISH or with molecular methods.

What are we looking for with the molecular analysis for FIP1L1-PDGFRA fusion gene? RT-PCR analysis of FIP1L1-PDGFRA fusion gene is more sensitive than FISH is the greater sensitivity of the method which allows the detection of the fusion gene even if the number of positive cells is low.

What are we looking for with the molecular analysis for Wilms tumor (WT) gene? RT-PCR on bone marrow or peripheral blood for WT1 can help to differentiate secondary or reactive eosinophilia (low levels of WT1) from idiopathic hypereosinophilia (Hyper Eosinophilic Syndrome) and chronic eosinophilic leukemia (high levels of WT1).

Have a look at the next page to once again review the cytogenetic abnormalities that we are trying to define in people with primary (clonal) eosinophilia!

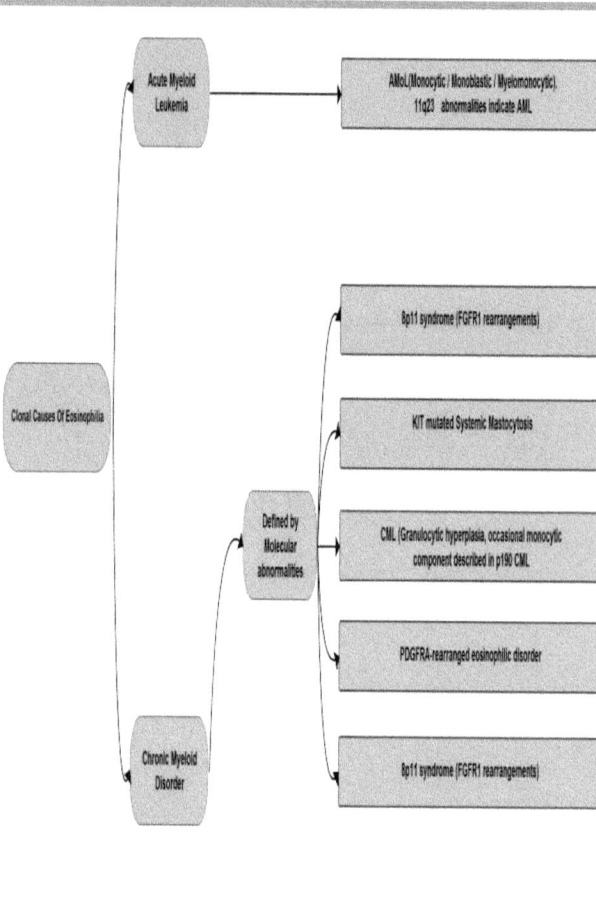

So once again. When we are evaluating a patient with eosinophilia we need to make sure they don't have a primary (clonal) disorder. We are going to check the following tests.

-Bone marrow aspirate and biopsy

-Cytogenetics on bone marrow aspirates.

-Peripheral blood for molecular analysis for FIP1L1-PDGFRA fusion gene.

-Peripheral blood for molecular analysis for Wilms tumor (WT) gene.

-Peripheral blood for evaluation of tryptase and decreased erythropoietin as well as demonstration of JAK2 which could indicate presence of a myeloproliferative disorders.

Lets think about the big picture again. We have primary (clonal), secondary (reactive) and idiopathic eosinophilia. Have a look at the next page.

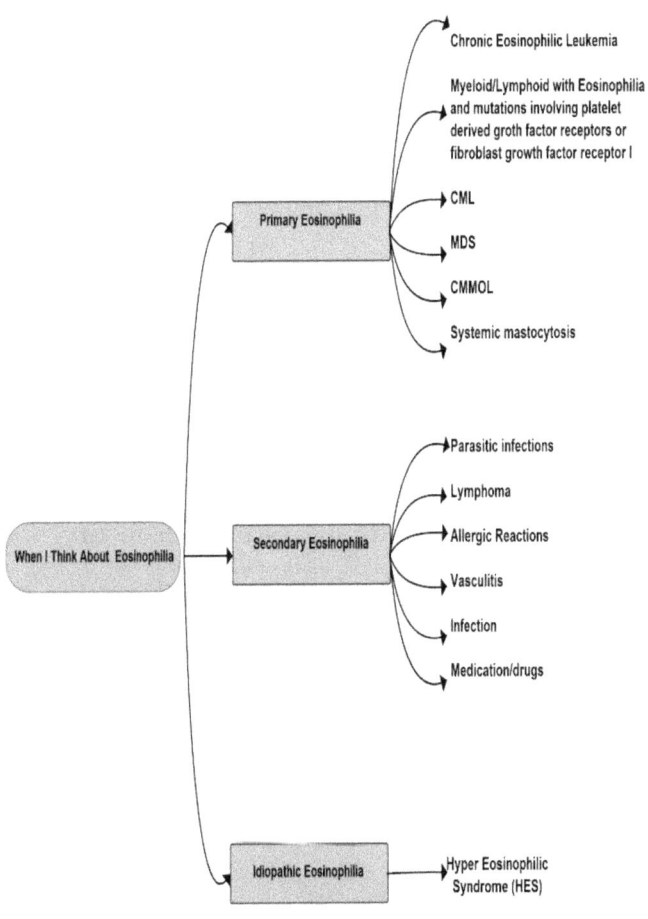

When I Think About Eosinophilia

Primary Eosinophilia
- Chronic Eosinophilic Leukemia
- Myeloid/Lymphoid with Eosinophilia and mutations involving platelet derived groth factor receptors or fibroblast growth factor receptor I
- CML
- MDS
- CMMOL
- Systemic mastocytosis

Secondary Eosinophilia
- Parasitic infections
- Lymphoma
- Allergic Reactions
- Vasculitis
- Infection
- Medication/drugs

Idiopathic Eosinophilia
- Hyper Eosinophilic Syndrome (HES)

Let us think about secondary (reactive) eosinophilia!

Here is a chart outlining various secondary (reactive) causes of eosinophilia.

Eosinophilia

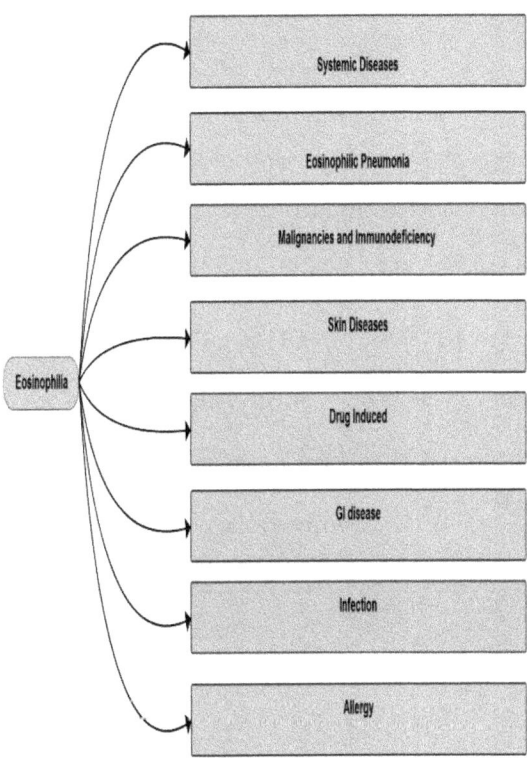

The classic concern in someone with eosinophilia is to make sure that they don't have a parasite. Parasites are a cause of secondary (reactive) eosinophilia. Have a look a the most common parasites that cause eosinophilia.

Which types of parasites can cause Eosinophilia?

-Helminth infections are considered the classic parasitic cause of eosinophilia.

-Ectoparasites such as scabies and myiasis (infestation with fly larvae) can cause eosinophilia.

-Protozoa usually do not cause eosinophilia. The specific protozoa that can sometimes cause eosinophilia include isospora belli, dientamoeba fragilis and sarcocystis hominis.

What is a Helminthic parasitic infection?

Helminths are generally considered a parasitic worm. Many of these are found in soil. Typically the worms live in the intestine and release eggs into the feces. In areas of poor sanitation, the eggs contaminate the soil, water, and food. When the eggs are ingested, they mature into worms in the intestine.

The most common Helminth species that cause human infection are the roundworm (Ascaris lumbricoides), whipworm (Trichuris trichiura) and the hookworms (Necator americanus and Ancylostoma duodenale).

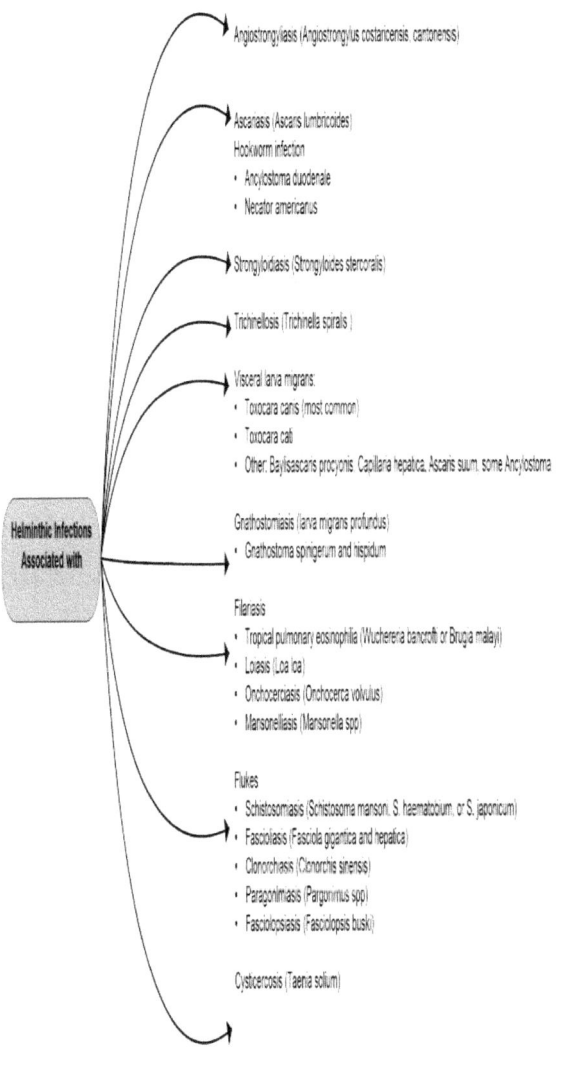

Helminthic Infections Associated with

Angiostrongyliasis (Angiostrongylus costaricensis, cantonensis)

Ascariasis (Ascaris lumbricoides)
Hookworm infection
- Ancylostoma duodenale
- Necator americanus

Strongyloidiasis (Strongyloides stercoralis)

Trichinellosis (Trichinella spiralis)

Visceral larva migrans
- Toxocara canis (most common)
- Toxocara cati
- Other: Baylisascaris procyonis, Capillaria hepatica, Ascaris suum, some Ancylostoma

Gnathostomiasis (larva migrans profundus)
- Gnathostoma springerum and hispidum

Filariasis
- Tropical pulmonary eosinophilia (Wuchereria bancrofti or Brugia malayi)
- Loaiasis (Loa loa)
- Onchocerciasis (Onchocerca volvulus)
- Mansonelliasis (Mansonella spp)

Flukes
- Schistosomiasis (Schistosoma mansoni, S. haematobium, or S. japonicum)
- Fascioliasis (Fasciola gigantica and hepatica)
- Clonorchiasis (Clonorchis sinensis)
- Paragonimiasis (Paragonimus spp)
- Fasciolopsiasis (Fasciolopsis buski)

Cysticercosis (Taenia solium)

How do we test for a parasite?

A stool sample will be sent for ovum and parasites. Serum testing can be done. A peripheral blood smear can sometimes identify parasites. At times the parasite is difficult to diagnose and a tissue biopsy may be needed.

Which helminthic infections can be diagnosed with serum antibody testing?.

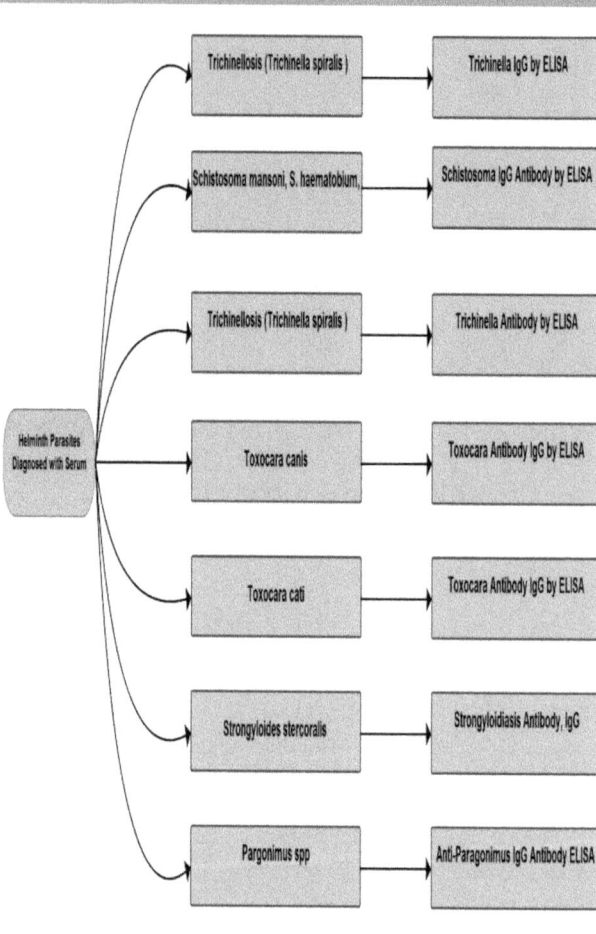

Which helminthic infections can be diagnosed
with stool testing for ovum and parasites?

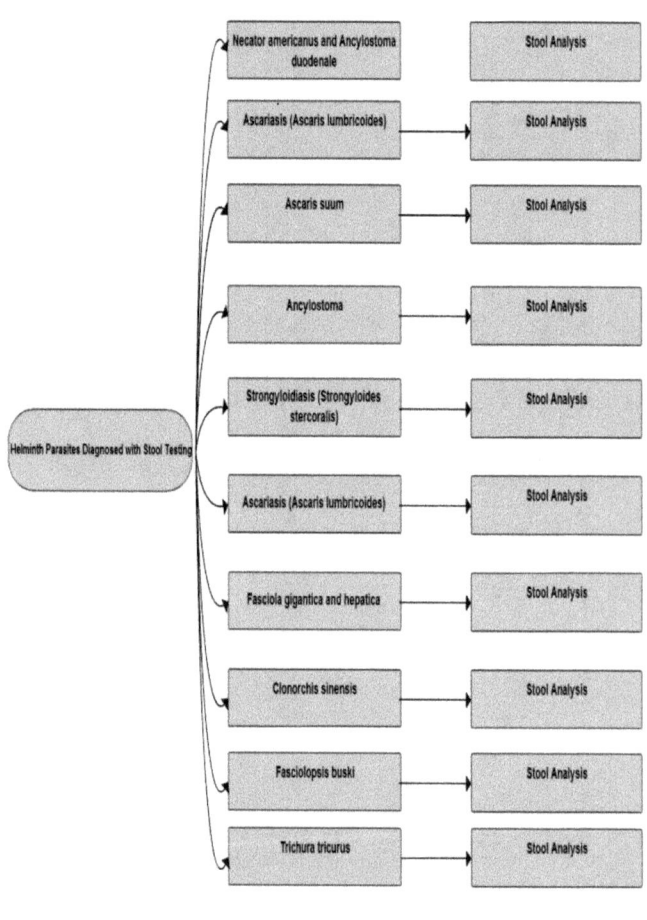

Which helminthic infections can be
diagnosed with visual analysis of
peripheral smear?

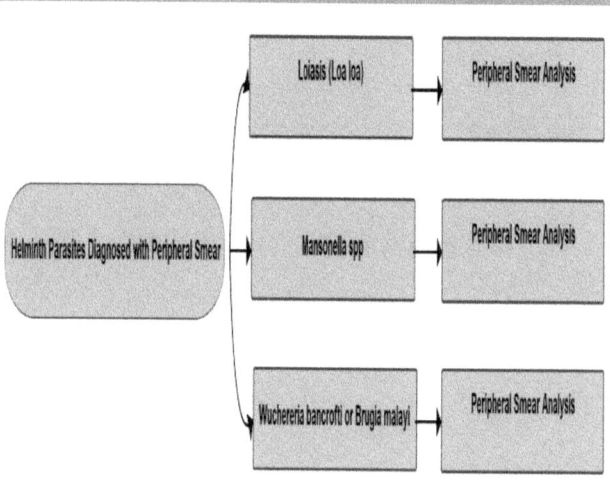

Helminth Parasites Diagnosed with Peripheral Smear

Loiasis (Loa loa) → Peripheral Smear Analysis

Mansonella spp → Peripheral Smear Analysis

Wuchereria bancrofti or Brugia malayi → Peripheral Smear Analysis

Which helminthic infections cannot be diagnosed with serum antibody testing, stool analysis or peripheral smear?

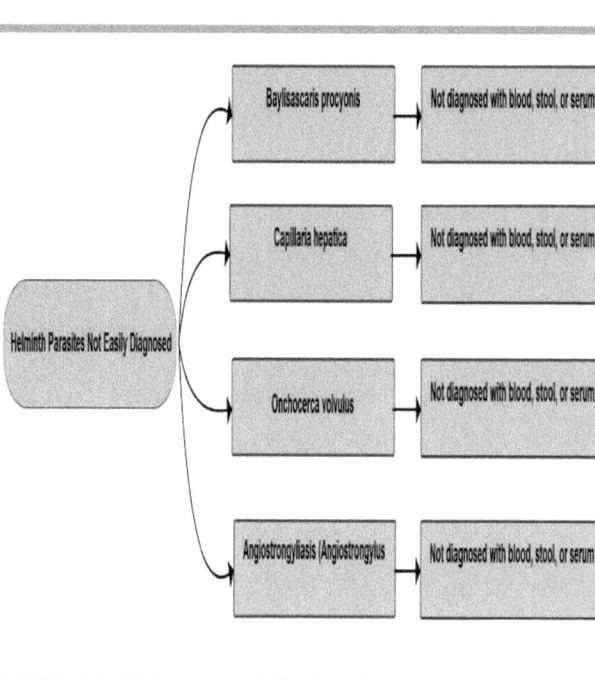

So let us review. How are you going to diagnose the most common Helminth species that cause human infection?

-The roundworm (Ascaris lumbricoides)

-The whipworm (Trichuris trichiura)

-The hookworms (Necator americanus and Ancylostoma duodenale)

The roundworm (Ascaris lumbricoides) is diagnosed with stool analysis.

The whipworm (Trichuris trichiura) is diagnosed with stool analysis.

The hookworms (Necator americanus and Ancylostoma duodenale) is diagnosed with stool analysis.

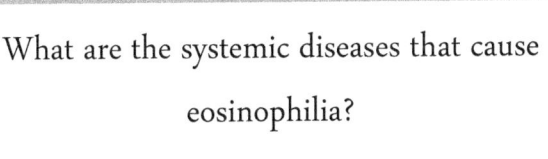

What are the systemic diseases that cause eosinophilia?

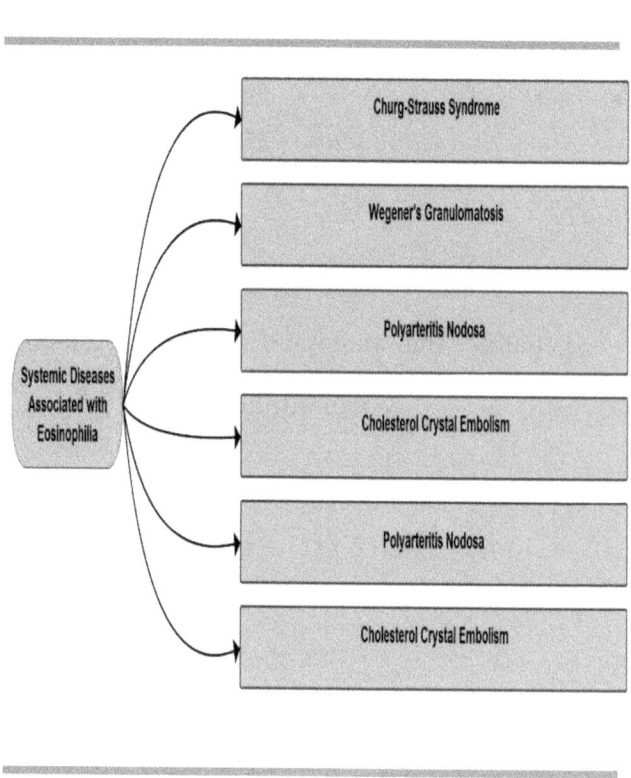

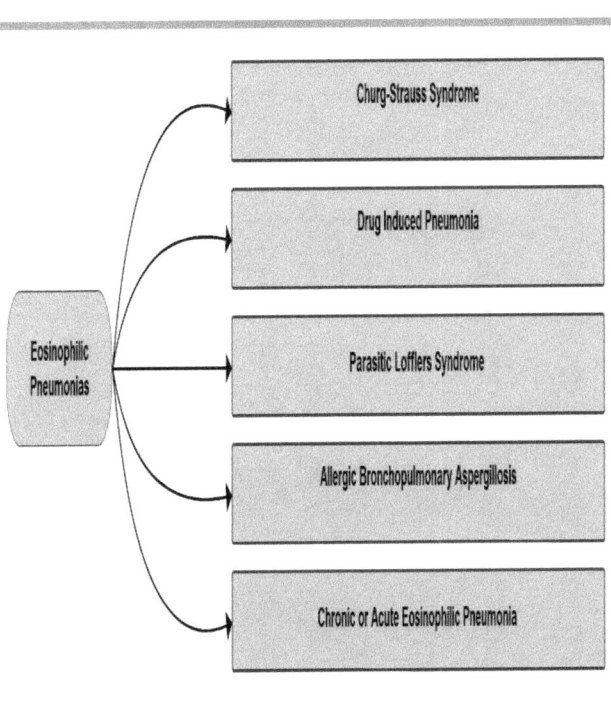

Eosinophilic Pneumonias

- Churg-Strauss Syndrome
- Drug Induced Pneumonia
- Parasitic Lofflers Syndrome
- Allergic Bronchopulmonary Aspergillosis
- Chronic or Acute Eosinophilic Pneumonia

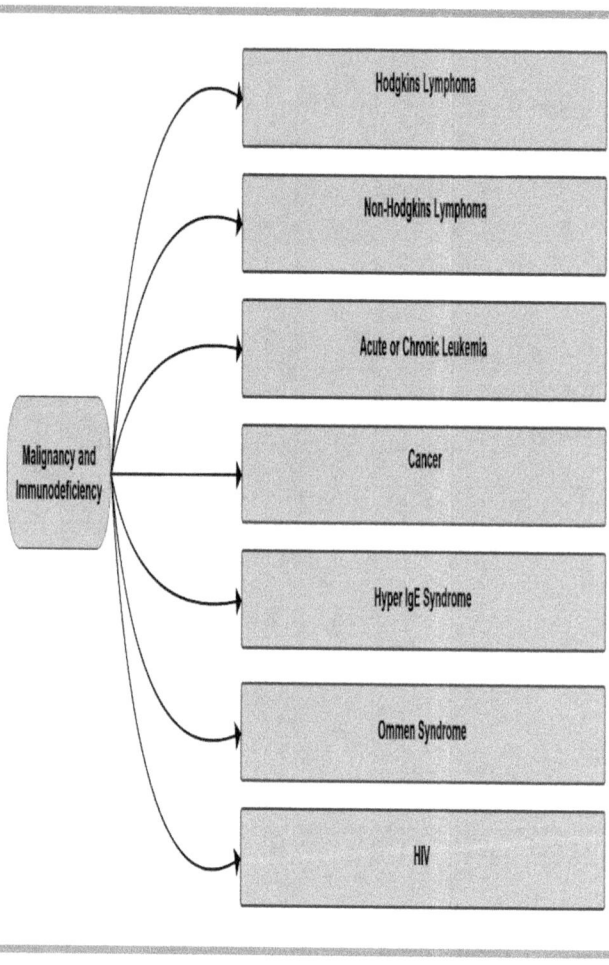

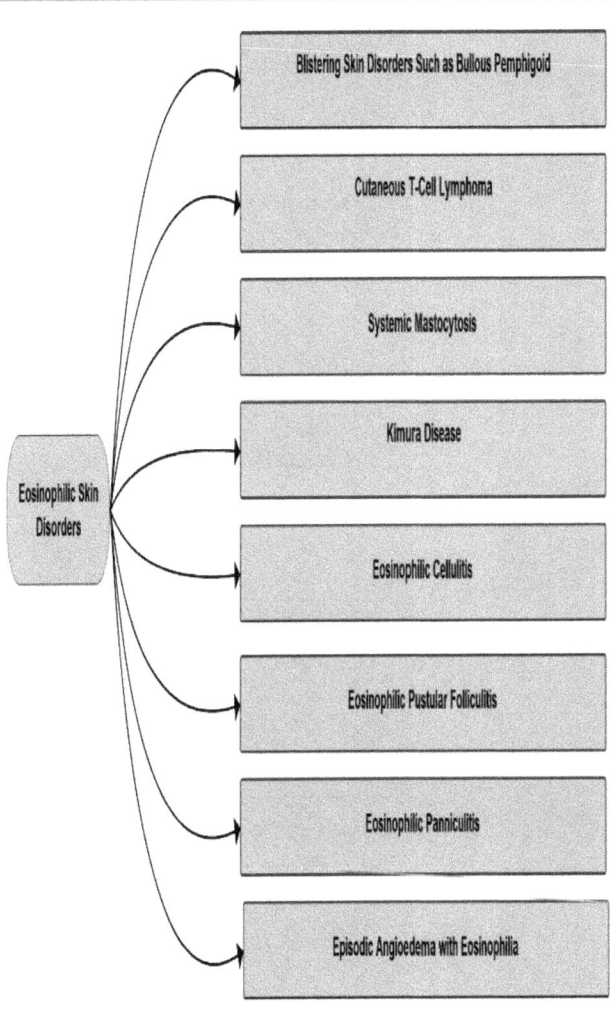

Eosinophilic Skin Disorders

- Blistering Skin Disorders Such as Bullous Pemphigoid
- Cutaneous T-Cell Lymphoma
- Systemic Mastocytosis
- Kimura Disease
- Eosinophilic Cellulitis
- Eosinophilic Pustular Folliculitis
- Eosinophilic Panniculitis
- Episodic Angioedema with Eosinophilia

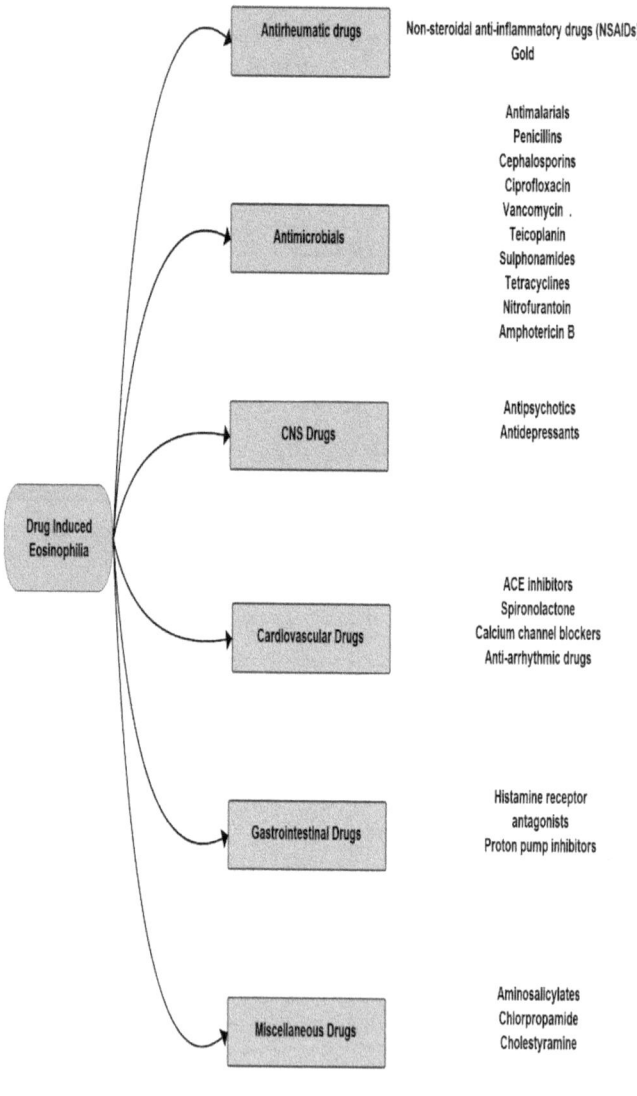

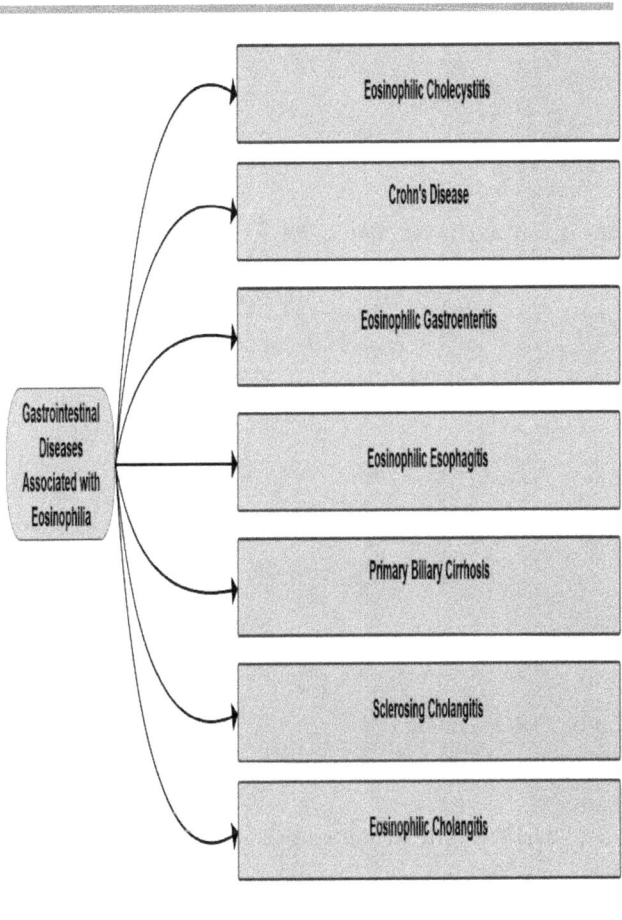

This concludes Eosinophilia: Fast Focus Study Guide

Search Amazon Kindle books to find other study guides written by

JT Thomas, MD

Internal Medicine Study Guide

Hematology Study Guide

Medical Oncology Study Guide

Cardiology Study Guide

Multiple Myeloma Study Guide

Differential Diagnosis Study Guide

Rheumatology Study Guide

Cancer Study Guide